The Carb Cycling Solution:

Maximize Weight Loss with a Powerful Meal Plan

TABLE OF CONTENTS

Introduction

In today's world, where obesity rates are on the rise and weight loss seems to be an elusive goal for many, it has become increasingly important to have a well-designed meal plan that can effectively aid in shedding those extra pounds. Weight loss is not just about restricting calories or following a generic diet; it requires a strategic approach tailored to individual needs. This is where carb cycling comes into play.

Carb cycling, a method that strategically alternates between high and low carbohydrate intake, has gained significant attention in the realm of weight loss and body transformation. By manipulating carbohydrate consumption, carb cycling harnesses the body's natural metabolic processes, optimizing fat burning and muscle recovery. The results? A powerful solution for maximizing weight loss and achieving a leaner, healthier physique.

The purpose of this book, "The Carb Cycling Solution: Maximize Weight Loss with a Powerful Meal Plan," is to provide you with a comprehensive understanding of carb cycling and guide you in implementing an effective meal plan tailored to your goals and preferences. Through the pages of this book, you will gain insights into the science behind carb cycling, learn how to design a personalized meal plan, and discover strategies to overcome challenges and maintain long-term success.

With the abundance of conflicting information available on weight loss and dieting, it can be overwhelming to determine the most effective approach. That's why we have compiled the latest research and practical strategies to help you navigate through the noise and embark on a journey towards sustainable weight loss.

Whether you are just starting your weight loss journey or have hit a plateau and are seeking a fresh approach, "The Carb Cycling Solution" will equip you with the knowledge and tools necessary to transform your body and achieve your weight loss goals. Get ready to unleash the power of carb cycling and embark on a life-changing adventure towards a healthier, fitter you.

Understanding Carb Cycling

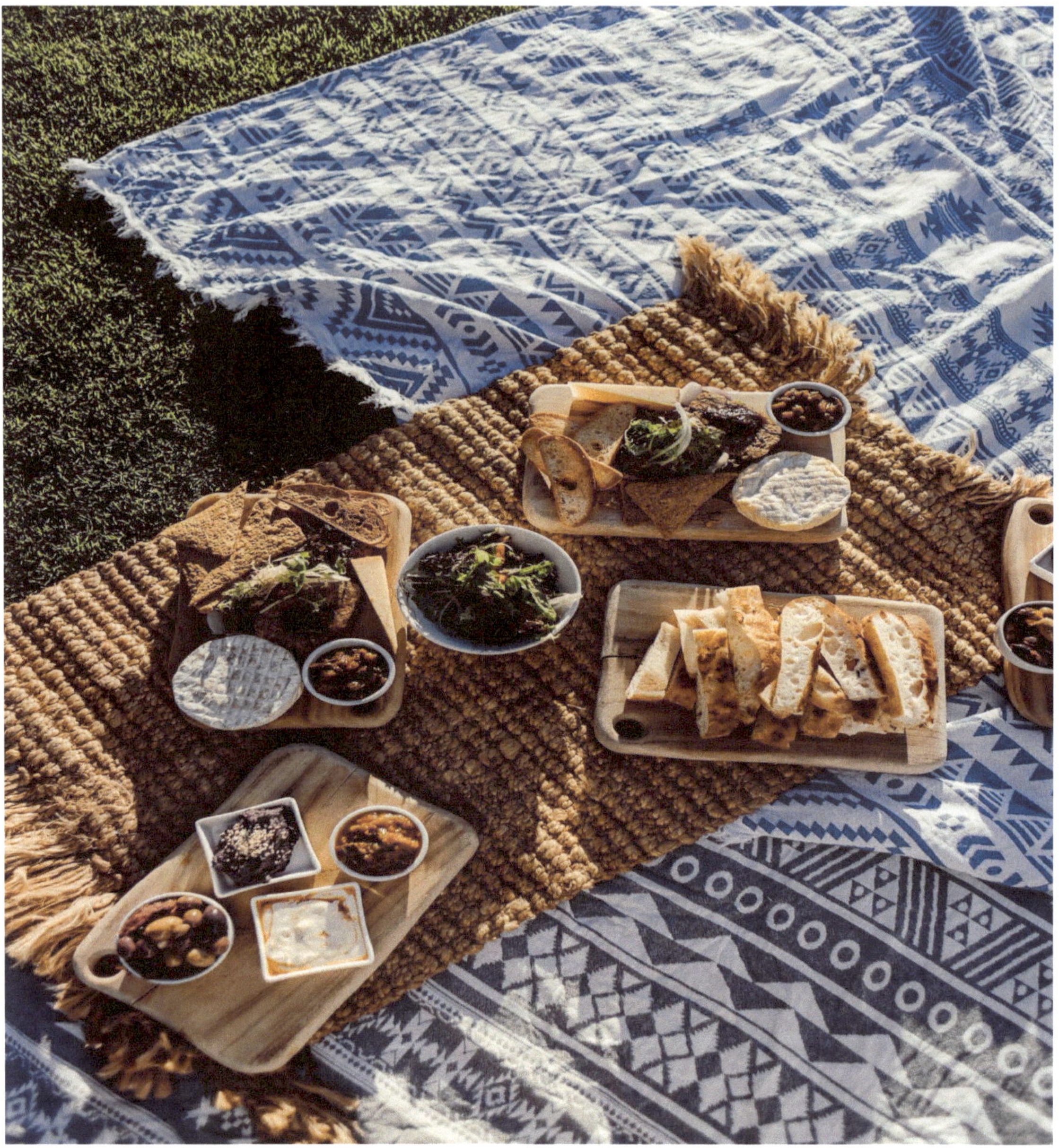

A. Definition and Concept of Carb Cycling

Carb cycling is a dietary approach that involves strategically alternating between high and low carbohydrate intake on different days or throughout the week. It is based on the principle that our bodies respond differently to varying levels of carbohydrate consumption, allowing us to optimize weight loss and muscle development. The concept of carb cycling revolves around the manipulation of carbohydrate intake to achieve specific metabolic responses and maximize results.

B. How Carb Cycling Affects the Body's Metabolism and Insulin Levels

Carb cycling has a profound impact on the body's metabolism and insulin levels. When we consume carbohydrates, they are broken down into glucose, which triggers the release of insulin, a hormone that regulates blood sugar levels. During high-carb days, the increased carbohydrate intake stimulates insulin production, promoting muscle glycogen storage and enhancing energy for physical activity. On low-carb days, insulin levels decrease, forcing the body to rely on stored fat for fuel, thereby promoting fat burning and weight loss.

By alternating between high and low carbohydrate days, carb cycling helps regulate insulin levels, prevent insulin resistance, and maintain a balanced metabolism. This cycling effect encourages the body to efficiently utilize carbohydrates for energy while also tapping into stored fat reserves.

C. Different Approaches to Carb Cycling (e.g., High-Low, Moderate-Low, Weekly Cycling)

There are various approaches to carb cycling, each offering different patterns of high and low carbohydrate intake. Some popular methods include:

High-Low Carb Cycling: This approach alternates between high-carb days, where the majority of calories come from carbohydrates, and low-carb days, where carbohydrate intake is significantly reduced. This cycling allows for muscle glycogen replenishment on high-carb days and fat burning on low-carb days.

Moderate-Low Carb Cycling: With this approach, carbohydrate intake is moderate on most days, followed by one or two consecutive days of low carbohydrate intake. This method strikes a balance between muscle recovery and fat burning while still providing a steady supply of energy for physical activity.

Weekly Carb Cycling: In this approach, the entire week is divided into different carbohydrate intake patterns. For example, the week might start with two high-carb days, followed by two low-carb days, and ending with moderate-carb days. This method provides flexibility and allows for customization based on individual preferences and goals.

D. Factors to Consider When Determining the Appropriate Carb Cycling Approach

When determining the most suitable carb cycling approach for you, there are several factors to consider:

Goals: Define your specific goals, whether it's weight loss, muscle gain, or overall body composition improvement. Different carb cycling approaches can be tailored to align with these goals.

Activity Level: Consider your activity level and energy requirements. If you engage in intense workouts or endurance training, you may need more carbohydrates to support performance and recovery.

Lifestyle and Preferences: Take into account your lifestyle and personal preferences. Some individuals may prefer more structure with specific high and low carb days, while others may find it easier to cycle their carbohydrate intake on a weekly basis.

Individual Response: Experiment and listen to your body. Everyone's response to carb cycling may vary, so monitor how you feel, your energy levels, and your progress to determine the optimal approach for you.

Understanding these factors will help you determine the most effective carb cycling approach that aligns with your goals, lifestyle, and preferences. In the next chapter, we will delve deeper into the science behind carb cycling and its impact on weight loss and body composition.

The Science Behind Carb Cycling

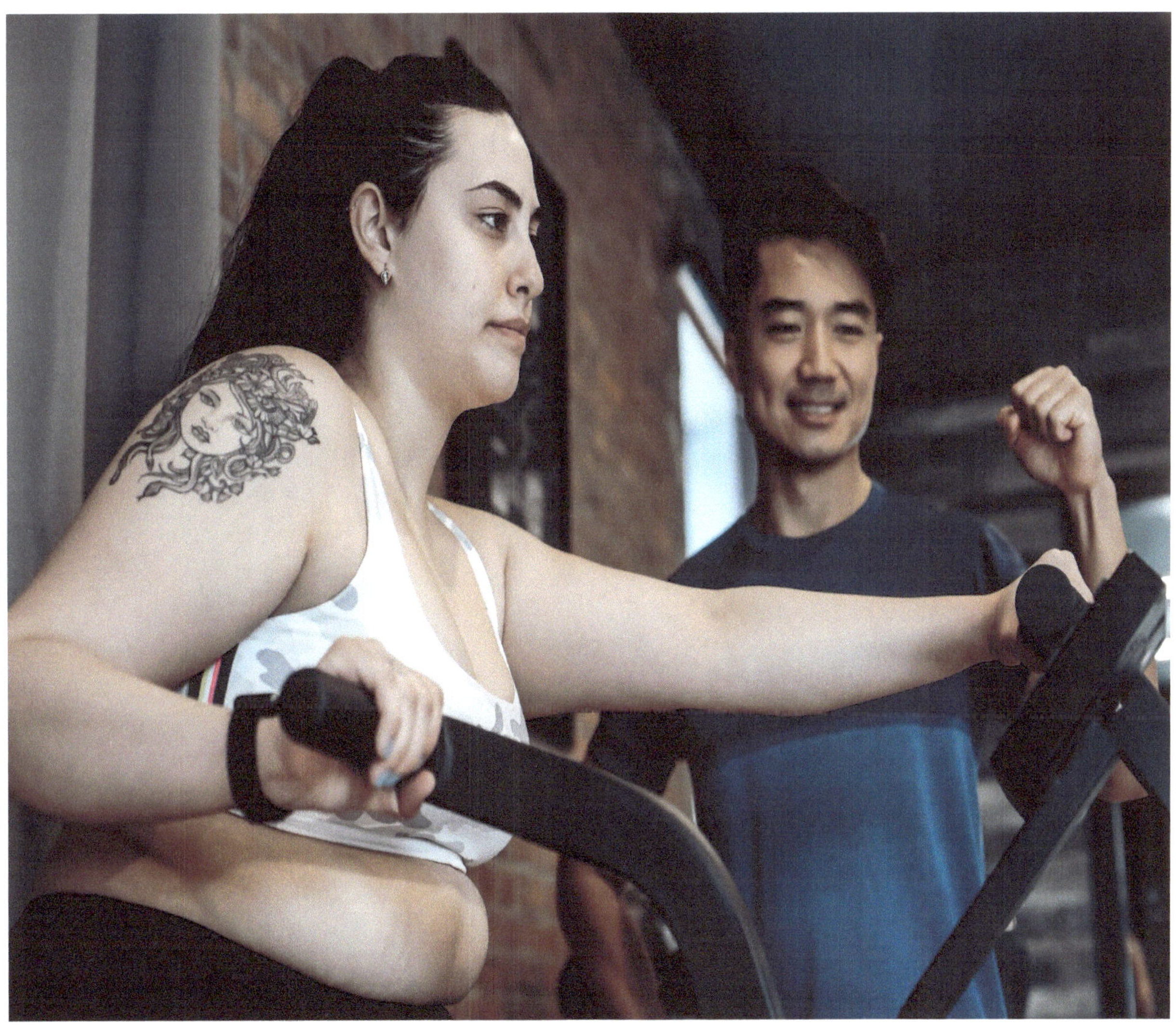

A. Role of Carbohydrates in the Body

Carbohydrates play a crucial role in providing energy to the body. When consumed, carbohydrates are broken down into glucose, which serves as the primary fuel source for various bodily functions, including brain function, muscle contraction, and cellular metabolism. Carbohydrates are stored in the body as glycogen in the muscles and liver, acting as a readily available energy reserve. Additionally, carbohydrates contribute to the synthesis of important molecules, such as nucleic acids and certain proteins.

B. Impact of Carbohydrates on Weight Loss and Fat Burning

The impact of carbohydrates on weight loss and fat burning is significant. When carbohydrates are consumed, insulin is released to facilitate the absorption of glucose into cells. Insulin also plays a role in fat storage. In a high-carbohydrate diet, where insulin levels remain consistently elevated, the body is more prone to storing excess carbohydrates as fat. This can hinder weight loss efforts.

However, restricting carbohydrate intake can lead to a decrease in insulin levels, promoting fat burning. During low-carbohydrate periods, the body's insulin sensitivity improves, allowing it to utilize stored fat as an energy source. This shift in fuel utilization from carbohydrates to fat can lead to accelerated fat loss and improved body composition.

C. Research Supporting the Effectiveness of Carb Cycling for Weight Loss

Numerous studies have examined the effectiveness of carb cycling for weight loss and have shown promising results. One study published in the Journal of the International Society of Sports Nutrition found that individuals following a carb cycling protocol experienced greater fat loss and preservation of lean muscle mass compared to those following a traditional continuous calorie restriction diet.

Another study published in the American Journal of Clinical Nutrition demonstrated that carb cycling can improve insulin sensitivity and promote fat loss, particularly in individuals with insulin resistance or metabolic syndrome.

Additionally, a study published in the Journal of Obesity showed that carb cycling may help prevent the metabolic adaptations that commonly occur with continuous calorie restriction, such as a decrease in resting metabolic rate and an increase in hunger hormones. This suggests that carb cycling may be a more sustainable and effective approach to long-term weight management.

D. How Carb Cycling Optimizes Hormone Levels for Better Results

Carb cycling can optimize hormone levels in the body, leading to improved weight loss outcomes. Insulin, as mentioned earlier, is a key hormone affected by carbohydrate intake. By manipulating carbohydrate consumption through cycling, insulin levels can be modulated, preventing insulin resistance and promoting better metabolic control.

Additionally, carb cycling can optimize other hormones involved in weight loss and body composition, such as leptin and ghrelin. Leptin is responsible for signaling satiety and regulating energy balance, while ghrelin stimulates hunger. Through carb cycling, these hormones can be regulated, helping to control appetite and prevent overeating.

Furthermore, carb cycling can influence the release of other hormones, such as growth hormone and cortisol, which play a role in muscle growth, recovery, and fat metabolism. By optimizing hormone levels through carb cycling, individuals can experience enhanced fat burning, muscle preservation, and overall improved body composition.

Understanding the scientific principles behind carb cycling provides a solid foundation for implementing this approach effectively. In the next chapter, we will guide you through the process of designing your personalized carb cycling meal plan, taking into account your goals, preferences, and nutritional needs.

Designing Your Carb Cycling Meal Plan

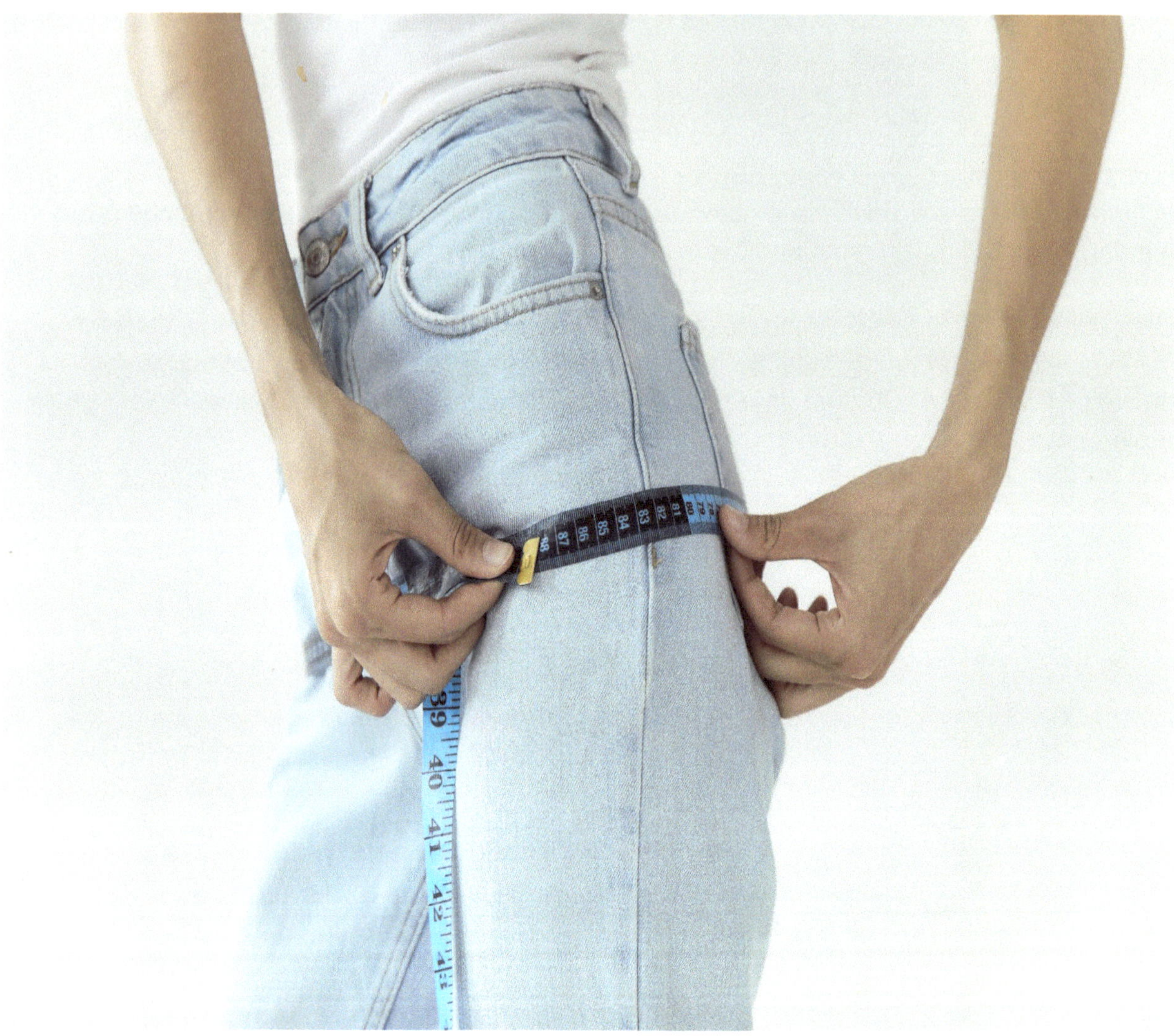

A. Assessing Your Current Dietary Habits and Goals

Before diving into designing your carb cycling meal plan, it's crucial to assess your current dietary habits and clearly define your goals. Take a close look at your eating patterns, food preferences, and any specific dietary restrictions or considerations. Identify areas where improvements can be made and determine your desired outcomes, whether it's weight loss, muscle gain, or overall health improvement. This self-assessment will serve as the foundation for creating a meal plan that aligns with your needs and preferences.

B. Determining Your Macronutrient Needs (Carbohydrates, Proteins, Fats)

To design an effective carb cycling meal plan, it's essential to determine your macronutrient needs. Macronutrients include carbohydrates, proteins, and fats, and their ratios in your diet play a significant role in achieving your goals.

Carbohydrates: Assess how your body responds to different levels of carbohydrate intake. Consider your activity level, energy requirements, and the cycling approach you intend to follow. On high-carb days, you may consume a higher percentage of calories from carbohydrates, while on low-carb days, your intake will be reduced.

Proteins: Determine your protein requirements based on factors such as your body weight, activity level, and goals. Protein is essential for muscle repair and growth, and it's recommended to consume an adequate amount to support your body composition goals.

Fats: Incorporate healthy fats into your meal plan, as they provide essential fatty acids and promote satiety. Choose sources such as avocados, nuts, seeds, and olive oil. Adjust the fat content based on your calorie needs and personal preferences.

Balancing the macronutrient ratios in your carb cycling meal plan will provide the necessary energy, support muscle growth and repair, and optimize metabolic function.

C. Creating a Calorie Deficit for Weight Loss

Weight loss is often achieved by creating a calorie deficit, which means consuming fewer calories than you expend. Calculate your daily calorie needs based on factors such as age, gender, weight, height, and activity level. Then, determine the appropriate calorie deficit for your weight loss goals.

During carb cycling, the calorie deficit can be achieved by adjusting the carbohydrate intake on low-carb days while maintaining an appropriate overall calorie intake. This strategic manipulation of carbohydrates helps optimize fat burning while still providing the necessary energy for physical activity and muscle recovery.

D. Structuring Your Meals and Incorporating Cycling Patterns

When designing your carb cycling meal plan, it's essential to structure your meals according to the chosen cycling pattern. Determine the frequency of high-carb and low-carb days based on your goals and preferences. For example, you might follow a two high-carb days followed by two low-carb days pattern, or a high-low cycling approach throughout the week.

On high-carb days, prioritize complex carbohydrates such as whole grains, fruits, and starchy vegetables. Include lean proteins, healthy fats, and ample amounts of fiber to support satiety and nutrient intake. On low-carb days, focus on non-starchy vegetables, lean proteins, healthy fats, and moderate portions of carbohydrates from sources like legumes and quinoa.

E. Sample Meal Plans for Different Carb Cycling Approaches

To help you get started, here are sample meal plans for different carb cycling approaches:

High-Low Carb Cycling:
High-Carb Day: Oatmeal with berries and almonds for breakfast, chicken breast with brown rice and steamed vegetables for lunch, salmon with quinoa and roasted asparagus for dinner.
Low-Carb Day: Scrambled eggs with spinach and avocado for breakfast, grilled chicken salad with mixed greens, cucumber, and olive oil dressing for lunch, baked cod with roasted Brussels sprouts and a side of quinoa for dinner.

Weekly Carb Cycling:
High-Carb Day: Whole wheat toast with avocado and scrambled eggs for breakfast, turkey and vegetable wrap with sweet potato wedges for lunch, grilled sirloin steak with roasted sweet potatoes and steamed broccoli for dinner.
Moderate-Carb Day: Greek yogurt with berries and almonds for breakfast, grilled chicken Caesar salad with whole grain croutons for lunch, baked salmon with quinoa and sautéed spinach for dinner.
Low-Carb Day: Vegetable omelet with a side of mixed greens for breakfast, grilled shrimp with zucchini noodles and marinara sauce for lunch, baked chicken breast with roasted cauliflower and a side of green beans for dinner.
These sample meal plans provide a starting point for structuring your carb cycling meal plan. Remember to adjust portion sizes and ingredient choices based on your individual needs and preferences. Experiment with different recipes and food combinations to keep your meals enjoyable and varied.

In the next chapter, we will discuss strategies for meal preparation, grocery shopping, and tracking your progress to ensure that your carb cycling journey is seamless and effective.

Maximizing Weight Loss with Carb Cycling

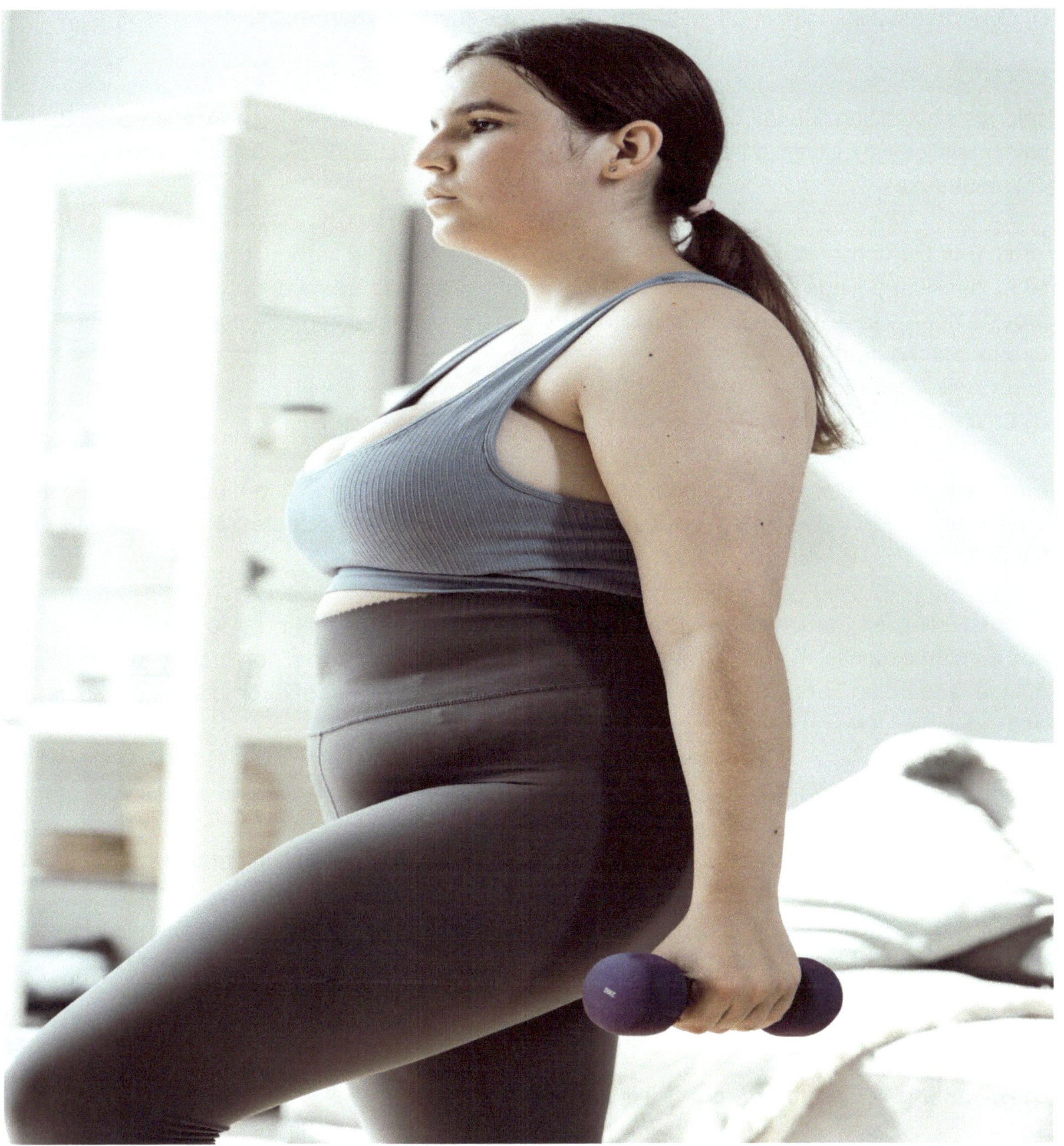

A. Strategies for Effective Fat Burning During Low-Carb Days

Low-carb days are a key component of carb cycling for maximizing weight loss. To optimize fat burning during these days, consider the following strategies:

Emphasize Protein and Healthy Fats: Increase your intake of lean proteins and healthy fats to promote satiety, preserve muscle mass, and support fat burning. Include sources such as chicken breast, fish, tofu, eggs, avocados, nuts, and seeds in your meals.

Focus on Non-Starchy Vegetables: Non-starchy vegetables are low in carbohydrates and calories while being rich in fiber and nutrients. Incorporate vegetables like broccoli, spinach, kale, cauliflower, zucchini, and bell peppers into your meals to add volume, fiber, and essential micronutrients.

Time Your Carbohydrate Intake: If you choose to consume some carbohydrates on low-carb days, consider timing them strategically. Consuming carbohydrates around your workouts can provide energy for exercise while still maintaining a lower overall carbohydrate intake throughout the day.

B. Leveraging High-Carb Days for Muscle Recovery and Performance

High-carb days are essential for replenishing glycogen stores, supporting muscle recovery, and enhancing performance during workouts. Consider the following strategies to make the most of these days:

Choose Complex Carbohydrates: Opt for complex carbohydrates that provide sustained energy and contain essential nutrients. Examples include whole grains, sweet potatoes, brown rice, quinoa, and fruits. These carbohydrates will provide the energy needed for intense workouts and aid in glycogen replenishment.

Prioritize Pre- and Post-Workout Nutrition: Consume a carbohydrate-rich meal or snack before and after your workouts to fuel your exercise and support muscle recovery. This can include a combination of carbohydrates and proteins to optimize the muscle-building process.

Adjust Caloric Intake: On high-carb days, you may need to adjust your overall calorie intake to accommodate the higher carbohydrate load. Monitor portion sizes and listen to your body's hunger and satiety cues to ensure you're consuming an appropriate amount of calories for your goals.

C. Balancing Your Nutrient Intake Throughout the Week

Maintaining a balance in your nutrient intake throughout the week is crucial for overall health and sustained weight loss. Consider the following tips to achieve a balanced approach:

Adequate Protein Intake: Ensure that you're consuming enough protein throughout the week to support muscle growth, repair, and satiety. Distribute protein-rich foods evenly across all your meals and snacks.

Healthy Fats: Include healthy fats in your meal plan consistently to support hormone production, satiety, and nutrient absorption. Choose sources such as avocados, nuts, seeds, olive oil, and fatty fish.

Micronutrient Variety: Incorporate a variety of colorful fruits and vegetables to ensure you're getting a wide range of vitamins, minerals, and antioxidants. Aim to include different types of produce throughout the week to maximize nutrient diversity.

D. Incorporating Exercise and Physical Activity to Enhance Weight Loss

While nutrition is a key component of weight loss, incorporating exercise and physical activity can significantly enhance your results. Consider the following tips:

Combination of Cardiovascular and Resistance Training: Include a combination of cardiovascular exercises (e.g., running, cycling, swimming) and resistance training (e.g., weightlifting, bodyweight exercises) to optimize fat burning, preserve lean muscle mass, and improve overall body composition.

Timing of Exercise: Consider scheduling your high-carb days around your most intense workouts to ensure you have sufficient glycogen stores for optimal performance.

Consistency and Progression: Stay consistent with your exercise routine and gradually increase the intensity and duration of your workouts over time. This progressive approach will help you challenge your body, increase calorie expenditure, and continue to see improvements in weight loss.

Non-Exercise Physical Activity: In addition to structured exercise, focus on increasing your non-exercise physical activity throughout the day. This can include activities like walking, taking the stairs instead of the elevator, gardening, or playing with your children. These small lifestyle changes can contribute to increased calorie expenditure and overall weight loss.

Listen to Your Body: Pay attention to how your body responds to different types of exercise and adjust accordingly. Some individuals may benefit from higher-intensity workouts, while others may find more success with moderate-intensity activities. Find what works best for you and listen to your body's needs.

Remember that weight loss is a gradual process, and consistency is key. Stay committed to your carb cycling meal plan, incorporate regular exercise, and monitor your progress. By implementing these strategies, you'll maximize your weight loss potential and achieve your desired goals.

Carb cycling recipes

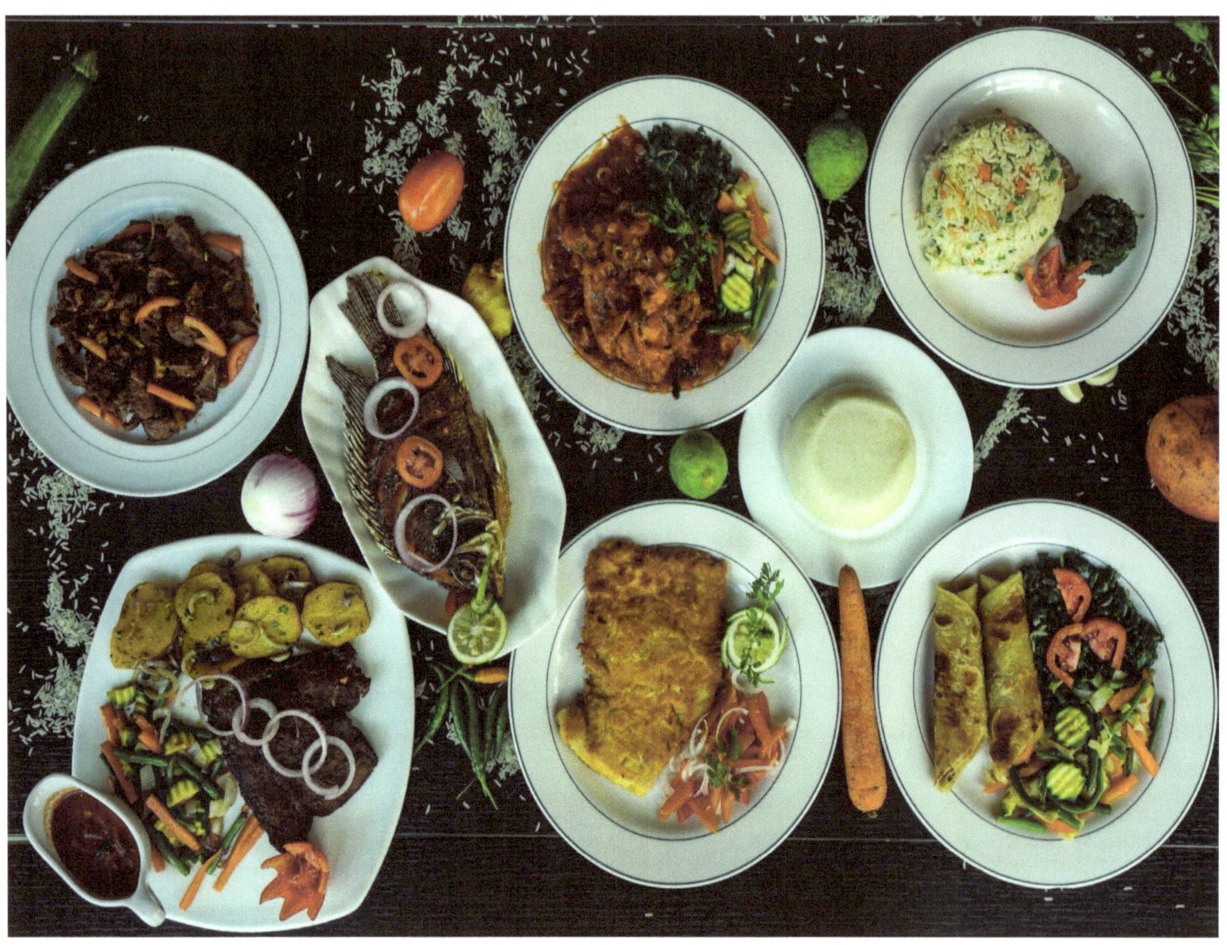

Breakfast recipes
1 High-Protein Omelette
Ingredients:
3 egg whites
1 whole egg
1/4 cup diced vegetables (bell peppers, onions, spinach)
Salt and pepper to taste
Instructions:
In a bowl, whisk the egg whites and whole egg together.
Add the diced vegetables, salt, and pepper to the egg mixture.
Heat a non-stick skillet over medium heat and pour the egg mixture into the pan.
Cook until the omelette is set and lightly browned, then flip and cook for an additional minute.
Serve hot.
Prep time: 10 minutes

2 Greek Yogurt Parfait
Ingredients:
1 cup Greek yogurt
1/4 cup mixed berries (blueberries, raspberries, strawberries)
1 tablespoon chia seeds
1 tablespoon honey or maple syrup (optional)
Instructions:
In a glass or bowl, layer Greek yogurt, mixed berries, and chia seeds.
Drizzle with honey or maple syrup, if desired.
Repeat the layers.
Serve chilled.
Prep time: 5 minutes

3 Quinoa Breakfast Bowl
Ingredients:
1/2 cup cooked quinoa
1/4 cup almond milk
1 tablespoon chopped nuts (almonds, walnuts, or pecans)
1 tablespoon dried cranberries
1 teaspoon honey or maple syrup
Instructions:
In a saucepan, warm the cooked quinoa with almond milk over medium heat.
Stir in the chopped nuts and dried cranberries.
Cook for 2-3 minutes, until heated through.
Drizzle with honey or maple syrup.
Serve warm.
Prep time: 10 minutes

4 Veggie Frittata
Ingredients:
3 eggs
1/4 cup diced vegetables (spinach, mushrooms, zucchini)
1 tablespoon chopped fresh herbs (parsley, basil)
Salt and pepper to taste
1 teaspoon olive oil
Instructions:
Preheat the oven to 350°F (175°C).
In a bowl, whisk the eggs together.
Add the diced vegetables, chopped herbs, salt, and pepper to the egg mixture.
Heat an oven-safe skillet with olive oil over medium heat.
Pour the egg mixture into the skillet and cook for 2-3 minutes until the edges set.
Transfer the skillet to the preheated oven and bake for 10-12 minutes until the frittata is cooked through.

Slice and serve.
Prep time: 15 minutes

5 Protein Pancakes
Ingredients:
1/2 cup oats
1/2 cup cottage cheese
2 eggs
1/2 teaspoon vanilla extract
1/4 teaspoon baking powder
Fresh berries for topping
Instructions:
Place oats, cottage cheese, eggs, vanilla extract, and baking powder in a blender.
Blend until smooth.
Heat a non-stick skillet over medium heat.
Pour 1/4 cup of the pancake batter onto the skillet.
Cook for 2-3 minutes until bubbles form on the surface, then flip and cook for an additional 1-2 minutes.
Repeat with the remaining batter.
Top with fresh berries and serve.
Prep time: 10 minutes

6 Avocado Toast with Egg
Ingredients:
1 slice whole grain bread
1/2 ripe avocado
1 poached or fried egg
Salt and pepper to taste
Optional toppings: sliced tomatoes, microgreens, hot sauce
Instructions:
Toast the slice of whole grain bread until crispy.
Mash the ripe avocado with a fork and spread it evenly onto the toast.
Top with a poached or fried egg.
Sprinkle with salt and pepper.
Add optional toppings, if desired.
Serve immediately.
Prep time: 10 minutes

7 Overnight Chia Pudding
Ingredients:
3 tablespoons chia seeds
1 cup unsweetened almond milk
1 tablespoon honey or maple syrup
1/4 teaspoon vanilla extract

Fresh fruit for topping
Instructions:

In a jar or bowl, combine chia seeds, almond milk, honey or maple syrup, and vanilla extract.
Stir well to ensure the chia seeds are fully immersed in the liquid.
Cover and refrigerate overnight or for at least 4 hours until the mixture thickens.
Stir again before serving.
Top with fresh fruit.
Enjoy chilled.
Prep time: 5 minutes (plus chilling time)

8 Cottage Cheese Bowl
Ingredients:
1 cup cottage cheese
1/4 cup granola
1/4 cup mixed berries
1 tablespoon almond butter or peanut butter
Instructions:
In a bowl, place cottage cheese as the base.
Sprinkle granola over the cottage cheese.
Top with mixed berries.
Drizzle almond butter or peanut butter on top.
Stir gently before eating.
Prep time: 5 minutes

9 Breakfast Quiche Cups
Ingredients:
4 large eggs
1/4 cup diced vegetables (spinach, bell peppers, onions)
1/4 cup shredded cheese (cheddar, mozzarella)
Salt and pepper to taste
Instructions:
Preheat the oven to 350°F (175°C) and grease a muffin tin.
In a bowl, whisk the eggs together.
Add the diced vegetables, shredded cheese, salt, and pepper to the egg mixture.
Pour the egg mixture evenly into the greased muffin tin.
Bake for 15-18 minutes until the quiche cups are set and slightly golden.
Allow them to cool slightly before removing from the tin.
Serve warm or at room temperature.
Prep time: 15 minutes

10 Berry Protein Smoothie
Ingredients:
1 cup unsweetened almond milk

1/2 cup frozen mixed berries
1 scoop protein powder (vanilla or berry flavor)
1 tablespoon almond butter
Ice cubes (optional)
Instructions:
1In a blender, combine unsweetened almond milk, frozen mixed berries, protein powder, and almond butter.
Blend until smooth and creamy.
If desired, add a few ice cubes and blend again until well incorporated.
Pour into a glass and serve chilled.
Prep time: 5 minutes

11 Sweet Potato Hash
Ingredients:
1 small sweet potato, peeled and diced
1/4 cup diced onions
1/4 cup diced bell peppers
2 slices turkey bacon, cooked and crumbled
Salt, pepper, and paprika to taste
1 teaspoon olive oil
Instructions:
Heat olive oil in a skillet over medium heat.
Add diced sweet potatoes, onions, and bell peppers to the skillet.
Season with salt, pepper, and paprika.
Cook for 8-10 minutes, stirring occasionally, until the sweet potatoes are tender.
Add the cooked and crumbled turkey bacon to the skillet.
Cook for an additional 2-3 minutes until everything is heated through.
Serve hot.
Prep time: 15 minutes

12 Protein-Packed Breakfast Wrap
Ingredients:
1 whole wheat tortilla
2 tablespoons hummus
2 slices turkey or chicken breast
1/4 cup mixed salad greens
2 slices tomato
Salt and pepper to taste
Instructions:
Spread hummus evenly over the whole wheat tortilla.
Layer turkey or chicken breast, mixed salad greens, and tomato slices on top of the hummus.
Sprinkle with salt and pepper.
Roll up the tortilla tightly.
Slice in half and serve.

Prep time: 5 minutes

13 Egg Muffins
Ingredients:
4 large eggs
1/4 cup diced vegetables (spinach, mushrooms, tomatoes)
1/4 cup crumbled feta cheese
Salt and pepper to taste
Instructions:
Preheat the oven to 350°F (175°C) and grease a muffin tin.
In a bowl, whisk the eggs together.
Add the diced vegetables, feta cheese, salt, and pepper to the egg mixture.
Pour the egg mixture evenly into the greased muffin tin.
Bake for 15-18 minutes until the egg muffins are set and slightly golden.
Allow them to cool slightly before removing from the tin.
Serve warm or at room temperature.
Prep time: 15 minutes

14 Green Smoothie Bowl
Ingredients:
1 frozen banana
1 cup spinach or kale
1/2 cup unsweetened almond milk
1 tablespoon almond butter
Toppings: sliced banana, granola, chia seeds
Instructions:
In a blender, combine frozen banana, spinach or kale, unsweetened almond milk, and almond
butter.
Blend until smooth and creamy.
Pour the smoothie into a bowl.
Top with sliced banana, granola, and chia seeds.
Serve chilled.
Prep time: 5 minutes

15 Blueberry Protein Pancake Bites
Ingredients:
1 cup oat flour
1 scoop protein powder (vanilla or berry flavor)
1 teaspoon baking powder
1/4 teaspoon salt
1/2 cup unsweetened almond milk
1/4 cup unsweetened applesauce
1/4 cup blueberries
Instructions:

Preheat the oven to 350°F (175°C) and grease a mini muffin tin.
In a bowl, whisk together oat flour, protein powder, baking powder, and salt.
Add almond milk and unsweetened applesauce to the dry ingredients and stir until well combined.
Gently fold in the blueberries.
Spoon the batter into the greased mini muffin tin, filling each cup about 3/4 full.
Bake for 12-15 minutes until golden brown and set.
Allow the pancake bites to cool slightly before removing from the tin.
Serve warm or at room temperature.
Prep time: 10 minutes

Lunch recipes
1 Grilled Chicken Salad
Ingredients:
Grilled chicken breast
Mixed greens
Cherry tomatoes
Cucumber
Red onion
Olive oil
Balsamic vinegar
Salt and pepper
Instructions:
Season the chicken breast with salt and pepper and grill it until cooked through.
Slice the grilled chicken breast into strips.
In a large bowl, combine mixed greens, cherry tomatoes, cucumber slices, and red onion.
Drizzle with olive oil and balsamic vinegar.
Add the grilled chicken strips on top.
Toss gently to combine. Serve.
Prep time: 15 minutes

2 Turkey Lettuce Wraps
Ingredients:
Ground turkey
Lettuce leaves
Bell peppers
Carrots
Green onions
Soy sauce (or tamari for gluten-free)
Sesame oil
Garlic powder
Ginger powder
Instructions:
In a skillet, cook ground turkey over medium heat until browned.
Add diced bell peppers, grated carrots, and sliced green onions to the skillet.
Season with soy sauce, sesame oil, garlic powder, and ginger powder.
Stir-fry until the vegetables are tender.
Spoon the turkey mixture onto lettuce leaves.
Roll up the lettuce wraps and secure with toothpicks if needed. Serve.
Prep time: 20 minutes

3 Shrimp Stir-Fry
Ingredients:

Shrimp, peeled and deveined
Broccoli florets
Bell peppers
Snap peas
Garlic cloves, minced
Ginger, grated
Soy sauce (or tamari for gluten-free)
Sesame oil
Red pepper flakes (optional)
Cauliflower rice (as a low-carb option)
Instructions:
Heat sesame oil in a large skillet or wok over medium-high heat.
Add minced garlic and grated ginger, and sauté for a minute until fragrant.
Add shrimp and cook until they turn pink.
Add broccoli florets, sliced bell peppers, and snap peas to the skillet.
Stir-fry until the vegetables are crisp-tender.
Season with soy sauce and red pepper flakes (if desired).
Serve over cauliflower rice or enjoy on its own.
Prep time: 25 minutes

4 Greek Quinoa Salad
Ingredients:
Cooked quinoa
Cherry tomatoes, halved
Cucumber, diced
Kalamata olives, pitted and halved
Red onion, thinly sliced
Feta cheese, crumbled
Fresh parsley, chopped
Lemon juice
Olive oil
Salt and pepper
Instructions:
In a large bowl, combine cooked quinoa, cherry tomatoes, cucumber, olives, red onion, feta cheese, and parsley.
Drizzle with lemon juice and olive oil.
Season with salt and pepper to taste.
Toss gently to combine. Serve chilled.
Prep time: 15 minutes

5 Chicken and Vegetable Skewers
Ingredients:
Chicken breast, cut into chunks
Bell peppers, cut into squares

Red onion, cut into wedges
Cherry tomatoes
Olive oil
Lemon juice
Garlic powder
Paprika
Salt and pepper
Instructions:
Preheat the grill or grill pan.
Thread chicken chunks, bell peppers, red onion, and cherry tomatoes onto skewers.
In a small bowl, mix olive oil, lemon juice, garlic powder, paprika, salt, and pepper to create a marinade.
Brush the skewers with the marinade.
Grill the skewers, turning occasionally, until the chicken is cooked through and vegetables are charred.
Remove from the grill and let them rest for a few minutes before serving.
Prep time: 20 minutes

6 Zucchini Noodles with Chicken Meatballs
Ingredients:
Zucchini, spiralized into noodles
Ground chicken
Onion, finely chopped
Garlic cloves, minced
Italian seasoning
Tomato sauce (check carb content for low-carb options)
Olive oil
Salt and pepper
Fresh basil (for garnish)
Instructions:
In a bowl, combine ground chicken, chopped onion, minced garlic, Italian seasoning, salt, and pepper.
Roll the mixture into small meatballs.
Heat olive oil in a skillet over medium heat.
Add the chicken meatballs and cook until browned on all sides and cooked through.
Remove the meatballs from the skillet and set them aside.
In the same skillet, add spiralized zucchini noodles and sauté for a few minutes until they are slightly tender.
Pour tomato sauce over the noodles and add the cooked meatballs.
Stir gently to combine and heat through.
Serve garnished with fresh basil.
Prep time: 25 minutes

7 Beef Stir-Fry with Broccoli

Ingredients:
Beef sirloin, thinly sliced
Broccoli florets
Red bell pepper, sliced
Mushrooms, sliced
Soy sauce (or tamari for gluten-free)
Sesame oil
Garlic cloves, minced
Ginger, grated
Red pepper flakes (optional)
Cauliflower rice (as a low-carb option)
Instructions:
In a bowl, marinate the beef slices with soy sauce, sesame oil, minced garlic, grated ginger, and red pepper flakes (if desired). Let it sit for a few minutes.
Heat sesame oil in a large skillet or wok over medium-high heat.
Add the marinated beef slices and stir-fry until browned.
Add broccoli florets, sliced red bell pepper, and mushrooms to the skillet.
Stir-fry until the vegetables are crisp-tender. Season with additional soy sauce if needed.
Serve over cauliflower rice or enjoy on its own.
Prep time: 25 minutes

8 Caprese Stuffed Chicken Breast
Ingredients:
Chicken breast
Mozzarella cheese, sliced
Tomato, sliced
Fresh basil leaves
Olive oil
Balsamic glaze
Salt and pepper
Instructions:
Preheat the oven to 375°F (190°C).
Slice the chicken breast lengthwise to create a pocket in the center.
 Stuff the chicken breast with slices of mozzarella cheese, tomato, and fresh basil leaves.
Season the chicken breast with salt and pepper.
Heat olive oil in an oven-safe skillet over medium-high heat.
Sear the stuffed chicken breast on both sides until golden brown.
Transfer the skillet to the preheated oven and bake for about 15-20 minutes or until the chicken is cooked through and the cheese is melted.
Remove from the oven and drizzle with balsamic glaze.
Let it rest for a few minutes before serving.
Prep time: 30 minutes

9 Egg Roll in a Bowl

Ingredients:
Ground turkey or pork
Coleslaw mix (shredded cabbage and carrots)
Onion, diced
Garlic cloves, minced
Ginger, grated
Soy sauce (or tamari for gluten-free)
Sesame oil Sriracha sauce (optional)
Green onions, chopped (for garnish)
Instructions:
In a large skillet, cook ground turkey or pork over medium heat until browned.
Add diced onion, minced garlic, and grated ginger to the skillet.
Sauté until the onions are translucent.
Add the coleslaw mix to the skillet and stir-fry until the cabbage is tender.
Season with soy sauce, sesame oil, and a dash of Sriracha sauce (if desired).
Stir to combine and cook for an additional minute.
Serve hot, garnished with chopped green onions.
Prep time: 20 minutes

10 Salmon with Roasted Vegetables
Ingredients:
Salmon fillet
Asparagus spears
Cherry tomatoes
Red onion, sliced
Lemon slices
Olive oil
Garlic powder
Dried dill
Salt and pepper
Instructions:
Preheat the oven to 400°F (200°C).
Place the salmon fillet on a baking sheet lined with foil.
Arrange asparagus spears, cherry tomatoes, and sliced red onion around the salmon.
Drizzle olive oil over the salmon and vegetables.
Season with garlic powder, dried dill, salt, and pepper.
Place lemon slices on top of the salmon.
Bake for about 12-15 minutes or until the salmon is cooked through and flakes easily with a fork.
Serve hot.
Prep time: 15 minutes

11 Greek Turkey Burgers with Tzatziki Sauce
Ingredients:
Ground turkey

Red onion, finely chopped
Garlic cloves, minced
Fresh parsley, chopped
Dried oregano
Salt and pepper
Whole wheat burger buns (or lettuce wraps for low-carb option)
Lettuce leaves
Tomato slices
Tzatziki sauce (store-bought or homemade)
Instructions:
In a bowl, combine ground turkey,
finely chopped red onion, minced garlic, chopped parsley, dried oregano, salt, and pepper.
Mix well until all the ingredients are evenly incorporated.
Shape the mixture into burger patties.
Preheat a grill or grill pan over medium-high heat.
Cook the turkey burgers for about 5-6 minutes per side or until cooked through.
Toast the burger buns if desired.
Place lettuce leaves and tomato slices on the bottom bun.
Top with a cooked turkey burger patty.
Drizzle tzatziki sauce over the patty.
Cover with the top bun and serve.
Prep time: 25 minutes

12 Cauliflower Fried Rice with Shrimp
Ingredients:
Cauliflower rice (fresh or frozen)
Shrimp, peeled and deveined
Frozen mixed vegetables (carrots, peas, corn)
Onion, diced
Garlic cloves, minced
Soy sauce (or tamari for gluten-free)
Sesame oil
Eggs, beaten
Green onions, chopped (for garnish)
Instructions:
In a large skillet or wok, heat sesame oil over medium heat.
Add diced onion and minced garlic, and sauté until the onion is translucent.
Add shrimp to the skillet and cook until they turn pink and are cooked through.
Push the shrimp to one side of the skillet and pour the beaten eggs onto the other side.
Scramble the eggs until cooked, then mix them with the shrimp.
Add frozen mixed vegetables and stir-fry until they are heated through.
Add cauliflower rice to the skillet and stir-fry for a few minutes until it's tender.
Season with soy sauce and mix well to combine.
Serve hot, garnished with chopped green onions.

Prep time: 20 minutes

13 Turkey Taco Lettuce Wraps
Ingredients:
Ground turkey
Taco seasoning (check for low-carb options)
Lettuce leaves
Tomato, diced
Avocado, diced
Red onion, diced
Fresh cilantro, chopped
Lime wedges
Salsa (optional)
Instructions:
In a skillet, cook ground turkey over medium heat until browned.
Add taco seasoning and follow the package instructions for seasoning.
Wash and dry lettuce leaves to use as taco shells.
Spoon the cooked turkey onto the lettuce leaves.
Top with diced tomatoes, avocados, red onions, and fresh cilantro.
Squeeze lime juice over the filling.
Serve with salsa on the side if desired.
Prep time: 20 minutes

14 Chicken and Vegetable Stir-Fry
Ingredients:
Chicken breast,Chicken breast, thinly sliced
Bell peppers, thinly sliced
Broccoli florets
Carrots, thinly sliced
Snow peas
Garlic cloves, minced
Soy sauce (or tamari for gluten-free)
Sesame oil
Red pepper flakes (optional)
Cauliflower rice (as a low-carb option)
Instructions:
In a large skillet or wok, heat sesame oil over medium-high heat.
Add minced garlic and sauté for a minute until fragrant.
Add sliced chicken breast and stir-fry until browned and cooked through.
Add bell peppers, broccoli florets, sliced carrots, and snow peas to the skillet.
Stir-fry until the vegetables are crisp-tender.
Season with soy sauce and red pepper flakes (if desired).
Serve over cauliflower rice or enjoy on its own.
Prep time: 25 minutes

15 Spinach and Feta Stuffed Chicken Breast
Ingredients:
Chicken breast
Spinach leaves
Feta cheese, crumbled
Sun-dried tomatoes, chopped
Garlic cloves, minced
Olive oil
Salt and pepper
Instructions:
Preheat the oven to 375°F (190°C).
Slice the chicken breast lengthwise to create a pocket in the center.
In a small bowl, combine spinach leaves, crumbled feta cheese, chopped sun-dried tomatoes, minced garlic, and a drizzle of olive oil.
Stuff the chicken breast with the spinach and feta mixture.
Season the chicken breast with salt and pepper.
Heat olive oil in an oven-safe skillet over medium-high heat.
Sear the stuffed chicken breast on both sides until golden brown.
Transfer the skillet to the preheated oven and bake for about 20-25 minutes or until the chicken is cooked through.
Remove from the oven and let it rest for a few minutes before serving.
Prep time: 30 minutes

Dinner recipes

1 Grilled Chicken with Roasted Vegetables

Ingredients:

4 boneless, skinless chicken breasts

2 cups mixed vegetables (such as bell peppers, zucchini, and broccoli)

2 tablespoons olive oil

Salt and pepper to taste

Fresh herbs for garnish (optional)

Instructions:

Preheat the grill to medium-high heat.

Season the chicken breasts with salt and pepper.

Brush the chicken breasts with olive oil.

Grill the chicken for 6-8 minutes per side or until cooked through.

Meanwhile, toss the mixed vegetables with olive oil, salt, and pepper.

Place the vegetables on a baking sheet and roast in the oven at 400°F (200°C) for 15-20 minutes or until tender.

Serve the grilled chicken with the roasted vegetables.

Garnish with fresh herbs if desired. Prep time: 25 minutes.

2 Shrimp Stir-Fry

Ingredients:

1 pound shrimp, peeled and deveined

2 cups mixed stir-fry vegetables (such as broccoli, snap peas, and carrots)

2 tablespoons low-sodium soy sauce

1 tablespoon sesame oil

1 tablespoon minced garlic

1 tablespoon minced ginger

Salt and pepper to taste

Instructions:

Heat sesame oil in a large skillet or wok over medium-high heat.

Add minced garlic and ginger and cook for 1-2 minutes until fragrant.

Add the shrimp and stir-fry for 2-3 minutes until pink and cooked through.

Add the mixed vegetables and cook for an additional 3-4 minutes until tender-crisp.

Stir in soy sauce and season with salt and pepper.

Serve hot. Prep time: 15 minutes.

3 Baked Salmon with Lemon Dill Sauce

Ingredients:

4 salmon fillets

2 tablespoons olive oil

Juice of 1 lemon

2 tablespoons chopped fresh dill

Salt and pepper to taste
Instructions:

Preheat the oven to 375°F (190°C).
Place the salmon fillets on a baking sheet lined with foil.
Drizzle the salmon with olive oil and lemon juice.
Sprinkle with chopped dill, salt, and pepper.
Bake for 12-15 minutes or until the salmon is cooked to your desired doneness.
Serve with lemon wedges and additional fresh dill if desired. Prep time: 10 minutes.

4 Turkey and Quinoa Stuffed Bell Peppers
Ingredients:
4 bell peppers (any color)
1 pound ground turkey
1 cup cooked quinoa
1/2 cup diced tomatoes
1/4 cup chopped fresh parsley
1 teaspoon dried oregano
1 teaspoon cumin
Salt and pepper to taste
Instructions:
Preheat the oven to 375°F (190°C).
Cut the tops off the bell peppers and remove the seeds and membranes.
In a large skillet, cook the ground turkey over medium heat until browned.
Stir in cooked quinoa, diced tomatoes, parsley, oregano, cumin, salt, and pepper.
Stuff the bell peppers with the turkey-quinoa mixture and place them in a baking dish.
Bake for 25-30 minutes or until the bell peppers are tender and the filling is heated through.
Serve hot. Prep time: 30 minutes.

5 Baked Chicken Parmesan
Certainly! Here's the continuation:
Baked Chicken Parmesan
Ingredients:
4 boneless, skinless chicken breasts
1 cup whole wheat breadcrumbs
1/2 cup grated Parmesan cheese
1 teaspoon dried basil
1 teaspoon dried oregano
1/2 teaspoon garlic powder
1/2 cup marinara sauce
1 cup shredded mozzarella cheese
Fresh basil leaves for garnish (optional)
Instructions:
Preheat the oven to 400°F (200°C).

In a shallow bowl, combine the breadcrumbs, grated Parmesan cheese, dried basil, dried oregano, and garlic powder.
Season the chicken breasts with salt and pepper.
Dip each chicken breast into the breadcrumb mixture, pressing lightly to adhere the crumbs.
Place the breaded chicken breasts on a baking sheet lined with parchment paper.
Bake for 20-25 minutes or until the chicken is cooked through and the breadcrumbs are golden.
Remove the chicken from the oven and spoon marinara sauce over each breast.
Sprinkle shredded mozzarella cheese over the marinara sauce.
Return the baking sheet to the oven and bake for an additional 5 minutes or until the cheese is melted and bubbly.
Garnish with fresh basil leaves if desired. Serve hot. Prep time: 30 minutes.

6 Cauliflower Fried Rice
Ingredients:

1 head cauliflower, riced (about 4 cups)
1 tablespoon sesame oil
1 cup diced mixed vegetables (such as carrots, peas, and bell peppers)
2 cloves garlic, minced
2 tablespoons low-sodium soy sauce
2 green onions, chopped
Salt and pepper to taste
Instructions:
Cut the cauliflower into florets and place them in a food processor. Pulse until the cauliflower resembles rice.
Heat sesame oil in a large skillet or wok over medium-high heat.
Add minced garlic and diced vegetables and cook for 3-4 minutes until the vegetables are tender-crisp.
Add the cauliflower rice to the skillet and cook for an additional 3-4 minutes until heated through.
Stir in soy sauce and season with salt and pepper.
Garnish with chopped green onions.
Serve hot. Prep time: 15 minutes.

7 Baked Cod with Lemon Butter Sauce
Ingredients:
4 cod fillets
2 tablespoons melted butter
Juice of 1 lemon
2 teaspoons chopped fresh parsley
Salt and pepper to taste
Instructions:
Preheat the oven to 400°F (200°C).
Place the cod fillets on a baking sheet lined with foil.

In a small bowl, whisk together melted butter, lemon juice, chopped parsley, salt, and pepper.
Drizzle the lemon butter sauce over the cod fillets.
Bake for 12-15 minutes or until the fish flakes easily with a fork.
Serve hot. Prep time: 10 minutes.

8 Turkey Meatballs with Marinara Sauce
Ingredients:
1 pound ground turkey
1/2 cup whole wheat breadcrumbs
1/4 cup grated Parmesan cheese
1/4 cup chopped fresh parsley
1 egg, lightly beaten
2 cloves garlic, minced
1 teaspoon dried basil
1 teaspoon dried oregano
1/2 teaspoon salt
1/4 teaspoon pepper
2 cups marinara sauce
Instructions:
Preheat the oven to 400°F (200°C).
In a large bowl, combine ground turkey, breadcrumbs, grated Parmesan cheese, chopped parsley, beaten egg, minced garlic, dried basil, dried oregano, salt, and pepper.
Mix well until all the ingredients are evenly incorporated.
Shape the mixture into meatballs, approximately 1 inch in diameter.
Place the meatballs on a baking sheet lined with parchment paper.
Bake for 20-25 minutes or until the meatballs are cooked through and browned.
While the meatballs are baking, heat the marinara sauce in a saucepan over medium heat until heated through.
Once the meatballs are done, transfer them to the saucepan with the marinara sauce and simmer for 5-10 minutes to allow the flavors to meld together.
Serve the turkey meatballs with marinara sauce over whole wheat pasta or zucchini noodles.
Garnish with additional grated Parmesan cheese and fresh parsley if desired. Prep time: 30 minutes.

9 Taco Salad
Ingredients:
1 pound lean ground beef or turkey
1 tablespoon olive oil
1 packet taco seasoning
4 cups shredded lettuce
1 cup diced tomatoes
1 cup canned black beans, rinsed and drained
1/2 cup sliced black olives

1/2 cup shredded cheddar cheese
1/4 cup diced red onions
1/4 cup chopped fresh cilantro
Salsa and Greek yogurt (optional) for serving
Instructions:
Heat olive oil in a skillet over medium heat.
Add the ground beef or turkey to the skillet and cook until browned.
Stir in the taco seasoning according to package instructions.
In a large salad bowl, combine shredded lettuce, diced tomatoes, black beans, black olives, shredded cheddar cheese, diced red onions, and chopped fresh cilantro.
Add the cooked ground beef or turkey to the salad bowl and toss everything together until well combined.
Serve the taco salad with salsa and Greek yogurt on the side if desired. Prep time: 20 minutes.

10 Lemon Herb Grilled Chicken
Ingredients:
4 boneless, skinless chicken breasts
Juice of 2 lemons
2 tablespoons olive oil
2 cloves garlic, minced
1 tablespoon chopped fresh thyme
1 tablespoon chopped fresh rosemary
Salt and pepper to taste
Instructions:
In a small bowl, whisk together lemon juice, olive oil, minced garlic, chopped fresh thyme, chopped fresh rosemary, salt, and pepper.
Place the chicken breasts in a shallow dish and pour the marinade over them, ensuring they are fully coated.
Cover the dish and refrigerate for at least 1 hour or overnight to allow the flavors to infuse.
Preheat the grill to medium-high heat.
Remove the chicken from the marinade, letting any excess drip off.
Grill the chicken for 6-8 minutes per side or until cooked through and juices run clear.
Remove from the grill and let it rest for a few minutes before serving.
Serve the lemon herb grilled chicken with your choice of sides, such as steamed vegetables or quinoa. Prep time: 10 minutes + marinating time.

11. Zucchini Noodles with Shrimp
Ingredients:
1 pound shrimp, peeled and deveined
4 medium zucchinis, spiralized
2 tablespoons olive oil
2 cloves garlic, minced
Juice of 1 lemon
1/4 teaspoon red pepper flakes

Salt and pepper to taste
Fresh parsley for garnish
Instructions:
Heat olive oil in a large skillet over medium heat.
Add minced garlic and cook for 1 minute until fragrant.
Add the shrimp to the skillet and cook for 3-4 minutes until pink and cooked through.
Stir in spiralized zucchini noodles and cook for 2-3 minutes until tender.
Drizzle lemon juice over the noodles and shrimp.
Season with red pepper flakes, salt, and pepper.
Toss everything together until well combined.
Garnish with fresh parsley.
Serve hot. Prep time: 20 minutes.

12. Veggie Quinoa Stir-Fry

Ingredients:
1 cup cooked quinoa
2 tablespoons olive oil
1 cup mixed stir-fry vegetables (such as broccoli, bell peppers, and snap peas)
2 cloves garlic, minced
2 tablespoons low-sodium soy sauce
1 tablespoon rice vinegar
1 teaspoon sesame oil
1/4 cup chopped green onions
Instructions:
Heat olive oil in a large skillet or wok over medium-high heat.
Add minced garlic and cook for 1 minute until fragrant.
Add mixed stir-fry vegetables and cook for 3-4 minutes until tender-crisp.
Stir in cooked quinoa and cook for an additional 2 minutes until heated through.
In a small bowl, whisk together soy sauce, rice vinegar, and sesame oil.
Pour the sauce over the quinoa and vegetables.
Stir well to coat everything evenly.
Garnish with chopped green onions.
Serve hot. Prep time: 15 minutes.

13. Baked Eggplant Parmesan

Ingredients:
1 large eggplant, sliced into rounds
1 cup whole wheat breadcrumbs
1/4 cup grated Parmesan cheese
2 teaspoons dried basil
2 teaspoons dried oregano
1/2 teaspoon garlic powder
1 cup marinara sauce
1 cup shredded mozzarella cheese

Fresh basil leaves for garnish (optional)
Instructions:
Preheat the oven to 375°F (190°C).
In a shallow bowl, combine breadcrumbs, grated Parmesan cheese, dried basil, dried oregano, and garlic powder.
Dip each eggplant slice into the breadcrumb mixture, pressing lightly to adhere the crumbs.
Place the breaded eggplant slices on a baking sheet lined with parchment paper.
Bake for 15-20 minutes or until the eggplant slices are golden and tender.
Remove from the oven and spoon marinara sauce over each slice.
Sprinkle shredded mozzarella cheese on top.
Return the baking sheet to the oven and bake for an additional 10 minutes or until the cheese is melted and bubbly.
Garnish with fresh basil leaves if desired.
Serve hot. Prep time: 30 minutes.

14. Grilled Salmon with Roasted Vegetables
Ingredients:
4 salmon fillets
2 tablespoons olive oil
Juice of 1 lemon
2 cloves garlic, minced
Salt and pepper to taste
4 cups mixed roasted vegetables (such as broccoli, cauliflower, and carrots)
Instructions:
Preheat the grill to medium-high heat.
In a small bowl, whisk together olive oil, lemon juice, minced garlic, salt, and pepper.
Brush the marinade onto the salmon fillets, coating them evenly.
Grill the salmon for 4-5 minutes per side or until cooked through.
While the salmon is grilling, roast the vegetables in the oven according to package instructions or until tender.
Serve the grilled salmon alongside the roasted vegetables.
Season with additional salt and pepper if desired.
Enjoy hot. Prep time: 20 minutes.

15. Stuffed Bell Peppers
Ingredients:
4 bell peppers (any color), tops removed and seeds removed
1 pound lean ground turkey or chicken
1 tablespoon olive oil
1 onion, chopped
2 cloves garlic, minced
1 cup cooked quinoa
1 can (15 ounces) diced tomatoes, drained
1 teaspoon dried oregano

1 teaspoon dried basil
1/2 teaspoon paprika
Salt and pepper to taste
1/2 cup shredded mozzarella cheese
Instructions:
Preheat the oven to 375°F (190°C).
Place the bell peppers in a baking dish and set aside.
In a large skillet, heat olive oil over medium heat.
Add chopped onion and minced garlic to the skillet and cook until softened.
Add ground turkey or chicken to the skillet and cook until browned.
Stir in cooked quinoa, diced tomatoes, dried oregano, dried basil, paprika, salt, and pepper.
Cook for an additional 2-3 minutes until heated through.
Spoon the turkey or chicken mixture into the bell peppers, filling them to the top.
Sprinkle shredded mozzarella cheese over the stuffed peppers.
Bake in the preheated oven for 20-25 minutes or until the peppers are tender and the cheese is melted and golden.
Remove from the oven and let them cool slightly before serving.
Enjoy hot. Prep time: 30 minutes.

Remember to adjust portion sizes and ingredients based on your specific carb cycling plan and dietary requirements. Enjoy your carb cycling dinner recipes!
Overcoming Challenges and Staying Consistent.

Overcoming Challenges and Staying Consistent

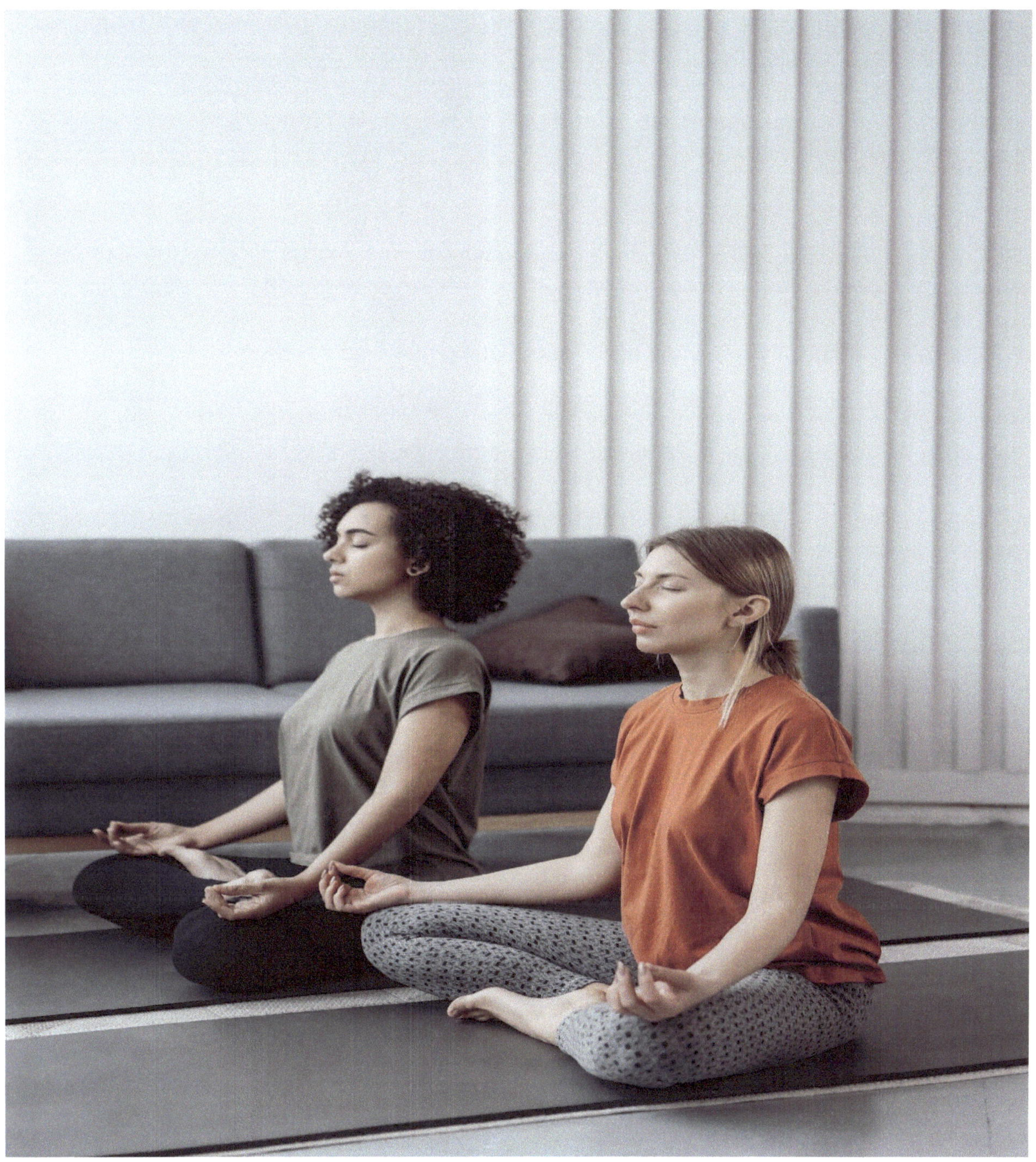

A. Dealing with Cravings and Managing Hunger during Low-Carb Days

During low-carb days, it's common to experience cravings and feelings of hunger due to the reduced carbohydrate intake. To overcome these challenges, consider the following strategies:

Increase Protein and Fiber Intake: Prioritize protein-rich foods and high-fiber sources to promote satiety and reduce cravings. Lean meats, legumes, leafy greens, and non-starchy vegetables can help you feel fuller for longer.

Stay Hydrated: Sometimes, thirst can be mistaken for hunger or cravings. Stay adequately hydrated by drinking water throughout the day. You can also try herbal teas or flavored water to add variety.

Plan for Snacks: Have healthy, low-carb snacks readily available to satisfy cravings. Opt for options such as nuts, seeds, Greek yogurt, cottage cheese, or vegetables with hummus.

B. Strategies for Social Situations and Dining Out While Carb Cycling

Navigating social situations and dining out can pose challenges when following a carb cycling meal plan. However, with some planning and strategies, you can stay on track:

Research Menus in Advance: Before going to a restaurant, review the menu online to identify carb-friendly options. Look for protein-based dishes with vegetable sides or ask for modifications to suit your needs.

Control Portion Sizes: Restaurants often serve larger portions, which can lead to overeating. Consider sharing a meal with a friend or packing half of your dish to-go to manage portion sizes.

Prioritize Protein and Vegetables: Opt for dishes that include lean proteins and non-starchy vegetables. Avoid or limit high-carb items like bread, pasta, and sugary sauces.

Be Mindful of Alcohol Consumption: Alcoholic beverages can be high in calories and carbohydrates. Limit your intake or choose lower-carb options like light beer, dry wines, or spirits with soda water and lime.

C. Tips for Meal Prep and Planning to Maintain Consistency

Meal prep and planning play a vital role in staying consistent with your carb cycling meal plan. Consider the following tips:

Set Aside Time for Meal Prep: Dedicate a specific day or time each week for meal prep. Prepare larger batches of protein, cook grains and vegetables in advance, and portion out meals for the upcoming days.

Use Portion-Controlled Containers: Invest in portion-controlled containers to pack your meals. This helps you manage portion sizes and makes it convenient to grab your pre-prepared meals on-the-go.

Plan Your Weekly Menu: Create a weekly menu and grocery list based on your carb cycling plan. This ensures you have all the necessary ingredients and helps prevent impulsive food choices.

Batch Cook and Freeze Meals: Make use of your freezer by preparing larger quantities of meals and freezing individual portions. This allows for variety and easy access to meals on busy days.

D. Tracking Progress and Making Adjustments When Necessary

Tracking your progress and making adjustments when needed is essential for long-term success. Consider the following tips:

Keep a Food Journal: Maintain a food journal to track your daily intake, including the types and quantities of food consumed. This helps you identify patterns, monitor portion sizes, and stay accountable.

Weigh Yourself Regularly: Regularly weigh yourself, preferably at the same time each week, to track your progress. Remember that weight fluctuations can occur due to various factors, so focus on long-term trends rather than day-to-day changes.

Assess Energy Levels and Performance: Pay attention to your energy levels and performance during workouts. If you feel consistently fatigued or notice a decline in performance, it may be an indication to adjust your carb cycling approach.

Consult with a Professional: If you're unsure about making adjustments or experiencing challenges with your carb cycling journey, consider consulting a registered dietitian or nutritionist. They can provide personalized guidance, help analyze your progress, and make appropriate recommendations.

Stay Flexible and Adapt: As your body changes and adapts to the carb cycling approach, you may need to make adjustments to keep progressing. Be open to experimenting with different cycling patterns, macronutrient ratios, or calorie levels to find what works best for your body and goals.

Celebrate Non-Scale Victories: Remember that progress goes beyond just the number on the scale. Celebrate non-scale victories, such as increased energy levels, improved sleep, better mood, or clothing fitting more comfortably. These indicators of progress can help keep you motivated and focused on the bigger picture.

Stay Consistent and Patient: Consistency is key when it comes to achieving long-term weight loss and health goals. Stick to your carb cycling meal plan, exercise routine, and lifestyle changes, even during challenging times. Remember that sustainable results take time, so be patient and trust the process.

By implementing these strategies, you can overcome challenges and maintain consistency throughout your carb cycling journey. Remember to be adaptable, seek support when needed, and stay focused on your goals. In the next chapter, we will provide additional tips for long-term success and lifestyle habits to support your weight loss efforts.

Maintaining Long-Term Success

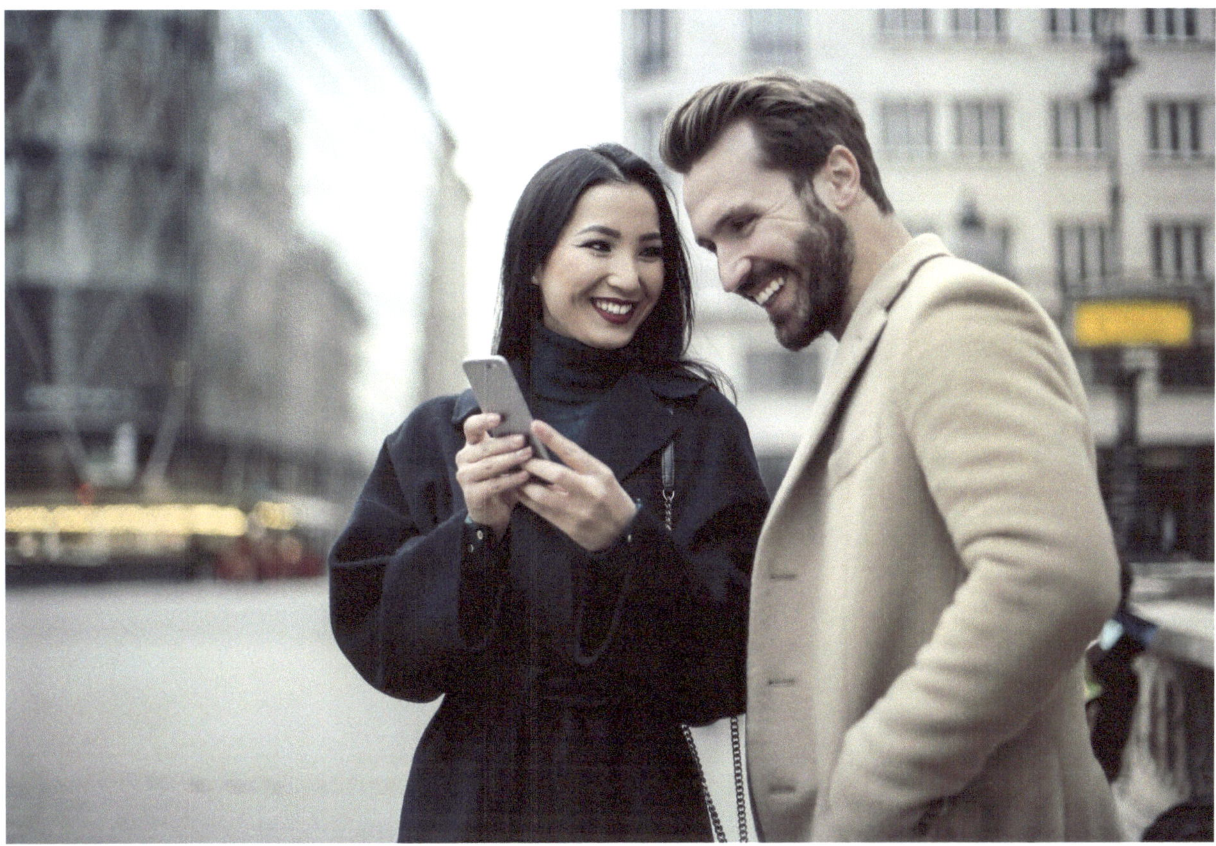

A. Transitioning Out of Carb Cycling and into a Sustainable Eating Plan

While carb cycling can be an effective short-term weight loss strategy, it's important to transition into a sustainable eating plan for long-term success. Consider the following strategies:

Gradual Adjustment: Slowly increase your carbohydrate intake over time, monitoring how your body responds. Pay attention to energy levels, mood, and changes in weight. Gradually reintroduce a wider variety of healthy carbohydrates while maintaining portion control.

Focus on Whole Foods: Emphasize whole, unprocessed foods in your eating plan. Incorporate lean proteins, fruits, vegetables, whole grains, and healthy fats. These nutrient-dense foods provide essential vitamins, minerals, and fiber for overall health and weight maintenance.

Portion Control and Mindful Eating: Practice portion control by being mindful of your hunger and fullness cues. Pay attention to portion sizes and listen to your body's signals to avoid overeating. Eating slowly and savoring each bite can help prevent mindless eating.

B. Strategies for Weight Maintenance and Preventing Rebound Weight Gain

Maintaining weight loss and preventing rebound weight gain requires ongoing effort and lifestyle changes. Consider the following strategies:

Regular Physical Activity: Continue to prioritize regular exercise and physical activity. Aim for a combination of cardiovascular exercises, resistance training, and activities that you enjoy. Engaging in at least 150 minutes of moderate-intensity exercise per week can help maintain weight loss and improve overall health.

Monitor Your Progress: Keep track of your weight and body measurements periodically to ensure you're staying within your desired range. If you notice any significant changes, reassess your eating habits and exercise routine to make necessary adjustments.

Set Realistic Goals: Set realistic weight maintenance goals that align with your body, lifestyle, and overall health. Focus on maintaining a healthy body composition, rather than striving for an unrealistic or unsustainable weight.

C. Incorporating Variety and Flexibility into Your Long-Term Eating Habits

To promote long-term adherence to a healthy eating plan, incorporate variety and flexibility into your meals. Consider the following tips:

Try New Recipes and Ingredients: Explore different recipes, cooking techniques, and cuisines to keep your meals interesting. Experiment with new vegetables, proteins, and whole grains to expand your palate and prevent food boredom.

Incorporate "Treat" Foods Mindfully: Allow yourself occasional indulgences or "treat" foods in moderation. Practice mindful eating by savoring these foods and being aware of portion sizes. This approach helps satisfy cravings without derailing your progress.

Plan for Social Events: Develop strategies for navigating social events while maintaining your healthy eating habits. Plan ahead by eating a balanced meal before attending, bringing a healthy dish to share, or focusing on the social aspects rather than solely on the food.

D. Tips for Staying Motivated and Focused on Your Weight Loss Goals

Staying motivated and focused on your weight loss goals can be challenging. Consider the following tips to stay on track:

Set Meaningful Goals: Continually reassess and set new goals that are specific, measurable, attainable, relevant, and time-bound (SMART). Having clear goals provides a sense of purpose and direction.

Find Support: Surround yourself with a supportive network of friends, family, or a weight loss community. Share your journey, seek advice, and celebrate achievements together. Having a support system can keep you motivated and accountable.

Reward Yourself: Acknowledge and celebrate your achievements along the way. Reward yourself with non-food-related treats, such as a spa day, new workout gear, or a fun activity that you enjoy.

Practice Self-Care: Prioritize self-care activities, such as getting enough sleep, managing stress, and engaging in activities that bring you joy and relaxation. Taking care of your overall well-being helps maintain a positive mindset and supports your weight loss journey.

Track and Celebrate Progress: Continue to track your progress beyond the number on the scale. Take note of non-scale victories, such as increased energy, improved fitness levels, or better sleep quality. Celebrate these milestones as they indicate your overall success.

Stay Educated: Stay informed about the latest research, nutrition guidelines, and strategies for healthy living. Keep learning about nutrition, exercise, and behavior change to enhance your understanding and make informed choices.

Visualize Success: Use visualization techniques to envision yourself reaching your weight loss goals. Imagine how you will look, feel, and the positive impact it will have on your life. Visualizing success can help you stay motivated and focused during challenging times.

Practice Resilience: Recognize that setbacks and plateaus are a normal part of the weight loss journey. Instead of becoming discouraged, view them as learning opportunities and a chance to reassess your approach. Practice resilience by bouncing back from setbacks and staying committed to your goals.

Remember, maintaining long-term success is not about achieving perfection but rather making sustainable lifestyle changes. Embrace the journey, be kind to yourself, and stay focused on your health and well-being.

In the final chapter, we will provide additional tips for staying motivated, managing setbacks, and embracing a lifelong commitment to a healthy lifestyle.

Conclusion

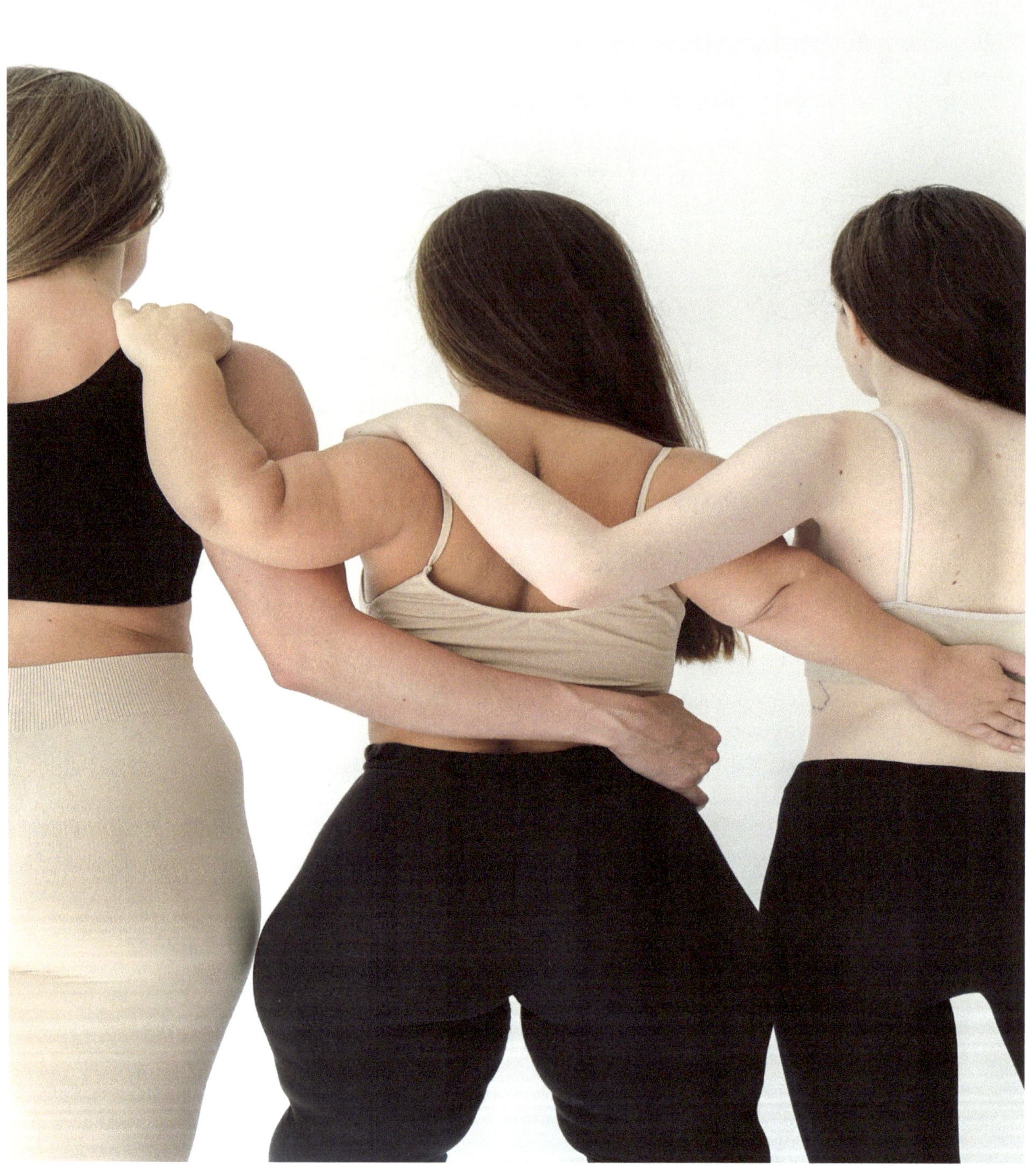

A. Recap of the Benefits and Effectiveness of Carb Cycling for Weight Loss

Throughout this book, we have explored the powerful weight loss strategy of carb cycling. We have learned how carb cycling can optimize your metabolism, improve insulin sensitivity, and enhance fat burning. By strategically manipulating your carbohydrate intake and cycling between high-carb and low-carb days, you can maximize weight loss while preserving muscle mass and supporting overall health.

Carb cycling offers a flexible and sustainable approach to weight loss, allowing you to enjoy the benefits of both low-carb and high-carb days. It provides variety in your meals, helps manage cravings, and optimizes nutrient intake for better results. Additionally, carb cycling supports hormonal balance, ensuring that your body is primed for efficient fat burning.

B. Encouragement for Readers to Implement the Carb Cycling Solution

I want to take this opportunity to encourage you, the reader, to implement the carb cycling solution and embark on your weight loss journey. Remember that change takes time and effort, but the rewards are worth it. By following the principles and guidelines outlined in this book, you have the tools and knowledge to achieve your weight loss goals.

I encourage you to embrace the flexibility of carb cycling, adapt it to your individual needs and preferences, and make it a sustainable part of your lifestyle. Trust the process, stay committed, and believe in your ability to succeed. Remember that progress is not always linear, but each step forward brings you closer to your desired outcome.

C. Final Thoughts and Resources for Further Support

As you continue your journey, it's important to seek ongoing support and resources to maintain your motivation and progress. Remember that you are not alone in this endeavor. There are various sources of support available to you, including:

Registered Dietitians and Nutritionists: Consult with a professional who specializes in weight loss and nutrition. They can provide personalized guidance, monitor your progress, and help you navigate any challenges that arise.

Online Communities and Support Groups: Join online forums, social media groups, or weight loss communities where you can connect with others on a similar journey. Share your experiences, seek advice, and celebrate milestones together.

Further Reading: Explore additional resources, books, and research on carb cycling, nutrition, and weight loss. Continually educate yourself to stay up-to-date with the latest information and strategies.

In conclusion, the carb cycling solution offers a powerful and effective way to maximize weight loss while enjoying the flexibility of different carb intake levels. By implementing the strategies outlined in this book and making sustainable lifestyle changes, you can achieve your weight loss goals and embark on a journey towards improved health and well-being.
Remember, your journey towards weight loss and improved health is unique to you. Embrace the lessons and insights shared in this book, but also trust your own instincts and listen to your

body. Adjust and customize the carb cycling approach to fit your preferences and lifestyle, ensuring long-term adherence and sustainability.

As you implement the carb cycling solution, keep in mind that achieving lasting results requires consistency, patience, and a positive mindset. Be kind to yourself along the way, celebrating both the big and small victories. Remember that setbacks and challenges are a natural part of any transformation process. Use them as opportunities for growth, learning, and self-reflection.

Maintaining a healthy lifestyle goes beyond just the physical aspect of weight loss. It encompasses nourishing your mind and soul as well. Practice self-care, cultivate positive habits, and surround yourself with a supportive environment that encourages your success.

Finally, I want to express my gratitude to you for choosing this book and embarking on this journey. I hope that the knowledge and insights shared within these pages empower you to achieve your weight loss goals and unlock your full potential. Remember, you have the power to transform your life and create the healthy, vibrant future you desire.

Wishing you health, happiness, and continued success on your carb cycling journey!